Chapter 1: Understanding Hand, Foot, and Mouth Disease

What is Hand, Foot, and Mouth Disease?

Hand, Foot, and Mouth Disease (HFMD) is a common viral illness primarily affecting young children but can also be observed in adults. Caused by enteroviruses, particularly the coxsackievirus, HFMD is characterized by fever, mouth sores, and a rash on the hands and feet. The disease is highly contagious and often spreads in childcare settings, making it essential for parents to be aware of its symptoms, transmission methods, and treatment options. While the illness usually resolves on its own within a week to ten days, understanding the nature of HFMD can help parents manage care effectively and reduce the risk of transmission.

The symptoms of HFMD typically begin with a mild fever, loss of appetite, and sore throat, which may evolve into painful lesions in the mouth and a rash that appears on the hands, feet, and sometimes the buttocks. These sores can make eating and drinking uncomfortable for affected children, highlighting the importance of dietary recommendations during the illness. Soft foods, cold beverages, and popsicles can provide relief from the discomfort while ensuring that the child stays hydrated and nourished. Parents should monitor their child's intake and seek medical advice if hydration becomes a concern.

Preventive measures in childcare settings play a crucial role in controlling the spread of HFMD. Good hygiene practices, such as regular handwashing with soap and water, sanitizing toys and surfaces, and keeping infected children away from group settings, can significantly reduce transmission rates. Educating caregivers and staff about the disease's symptoms and preventive strategies is vital in managing outbreaks in schools and daycare facilities. By fostering a culture of hygiene and awareness, parents can help protect not only their children but also the wider community.

While HFMD is generally mild and self-limiting, there can be complications, particularly in rare cases where the infection leads to viral meningitis or encephalitis. Parents should remain vigilant for any signs of worsening symptoms, such as high fever, persistent headache, or extreme lethargy. Understanding the potential complications associated with HFMD can empower parents to seek timely medical intervention when necessary. It is also important to note that adults can contract HFMD, often experiencing milder symptoms, yet the risk of transmission remains, making education and preventive measures equally relevant for all age groups.

Natural treatments and home remedies may provide additional comfort during recovery. Herbal teas, honey, and other soothing remedies can help alleviate symptoms and promote healing. However, parents should consult with healthcare professionals before introducing any new treatments. Resources such as educational pamphlets, community workshops, and online forums can provide further information, equipping parents with tools to navigate the challenges of HFMD effectively. By understanding the disease and its implications, parents can help their children recover more comfortably while minimizing the risk of spreading the infection.

Causes and Symptoms

Hand, foot, and mouth disease (HFMD) is primarily caused by enteroviruses, with the coxsackievirus A16 and enterovirus 71 being the most common culprits. These viruses are highly contagious and can spread through direct contact with an infected person's nasal secretions, saliva, or fluid from the blisters. Children are particularly susceptible due to their frequent close contact in settings like daycare centers and playgrounds. Understanding how the disease spreads is crucial for parents to implement effective preventive measures, such as reinforcing good hygiene practices and minimizing exposure during outbreaks.

Symptoms of HFMD typically begin with a mild fever, sore throat, and general malaise, which can be easily mistaken for other common childhood illnesses. Within a day or two, painful sores may develop in the mouth, along with a rash that appears on the hands, feet, and sometimes the buttocks. The sores in the mouth can make it difficult for children to eat or drink, leading to discomfort and potential dehydration. Parents should be vigilant for these signs and monitor their child's symptoms closely, as they can vary in severity and duration.

In terms of dietary recommendations during HFMD, it is vital to focus on soft, bland foods that are easy to swallow and gentle on the throat. Foods such as yogurt, applesauce, and smoothies can provide necessary nutrition while minimizing discomfort. Hydration is particularly important, and offering cold fluids can help soothe sore mouths. Avoiding acidic or spicy foods is advisable, as these can exacerbate the pain associated with mouth sores. Parents should aim to create a soothing eating environment to encourage their child to consume enough fluids and nutrition during recovery.

While most cases of HFMD resolve on their own within a week to ten days, complications can arise, albeit rarely. These may include viral meningitis or encephalitis, which require immediate medical attention. Parents should seek care if their child exhibits severe symptoms such as persistent high fever, extreme lethargy, or difficulty breathing. Being aware of these potential complications allows parents to act swiftly and ensure their child's health is monitored closely during the illness.

Preventive measures play a critical role in managing HFMD, especially in childcare settings where children are in close proximity. Regular handwashing, sanitizing surfaces, and avoiding shared items can significantly reduce the risk of transmission. Educating children about the importance of hygiene is also essential; simple practices such as covering coughs and sneezes can make a difference. Additionally, while there is no specific vaccine for HFMD, maintaining overall health and immunity through a balanced diet and appropriate vaccinations can help reduce the risk of infection and its complications.

How it Spreads

Hand, foot, and mouth disease (HFMD) is primarily caused by viruses from the enterovirus family, most commonly the Coxsackievirus A16 and Enterovirus 71. The disease is highly contagious and spreads easily among children, especially in settings like daycare centers and schools. Understanding how HFMD spreads is crucial for parents to take appropriate preventive measures. The virus is typically transmitted through direct contact with an infected person's saliva, blister fluid, or feces. This can occur during activities such as hugging, sharing utensils, or touching contaminated surfaces.

The virus can also spread through respiratory droplets when an infected person coughs or sneezes. Parents should be particularly vigilant during outbreaks in schools or childcare settings, as children often have close contact with one another. This close proximity increases the likelihood of transmission, particularly in communal areas such as playgrounds or shared classrooms. It is essential for parents to educate their children about the importance of personal space and hygiene, such as covering their mouths when coughing and avoiding sharing personal items.

In addition to direct contact, the virus can survive on surfaces for several hours, increasing the risk of indirect transmission. Commonly touched surfaces, such as toys, doorknobs, and bathroom fixtures, can harbor the virus and facilitate its spread among children. Regular cleaning and disinfecting of these surfaces can significantly reduce the risk of infection. Parents should implement routine cleaning practices in their homes and encourage daycare providers to maintain a strict cleaning schedule to minimize the spread of HFMD.

Another important aspect of the spread of HFMD is the asymptomatic carrier state. Some individuals may carry the virus without showing any symptoms, making it challenging to identify and contain outbreaks. This silent transmission can lead to unexpected cases, particularly in settings where children interact closely. Parents should be aware that even if their child appears healthy, they could still be spreading the virus to others. Vigilant monitoring for symptoms, even in the absence of overt signs of illness, is essential for controlling the spread of HFMD.

Preventive measures play a crucial role in controlling the transmission of HFMD. Parents should encourage frequent handwashing with soap and water, especially after using the bathroom and before eating. Additionally, limiting close contact with infected individuals and keeping sick children at home until they are fully recovered can help contain outbreaks. Educating themselves and their children about the disease, its transmission, and preventive practices can empower parents to effectively navigate the challenges posed by hand, foot, and mouth disease.

Chapter 2: Pediatric Care for Hand, Foot, and Mouth Disease

Recognizing Symptoms in Children

Recognizing the symptoms of hand, foot, and mouth disease (HFMD) in children is crucial for timely intervention and care. The initial signs typically manifest within three to six days post-exposure to the virus, which often includes the Coxsackievirus. Parents should be vigilant for a combination of symptoms that can help in identifying the disease early. The first indicators usually include a mild fever, sore throat, and reduced appetite. Observing these symptoms can prompt parents to monitor their child more closely for the development of additional signs.

As the illness progresses, the characteristic rash appears on the hands, feet, and inside the mouth. This rash often begins as small red spots that can evolve into painful blisters. The presence of these blisters in the mouth can lead to difficulty swallowing and increased irritability in children, making it particularly important for parents to ensure that their child remains hydrated. Recognizing these physical manifestations is essential in managing the child's comfort and preventing complications, such as dehydration.

In addition to the visible signs, parents should also be aware of behavioral changes that may accompany HFMD. Children may exhibit increased fussiness or discomfort, especially when eating or drinking, due to the painful sores in the mouth. These behavioral cues can be indicative of the severity of the illness and can guide parents in seeking medical advice. Monitoring a child's mood and activity levels can provide valuable insights into their overall condition and the effectiveness of any home remedies being applied.

A significant aspect of recognizing symptoms in children is understanding the potential for complications. While HFMD is generally mild, some children may experience more severe symptoms or secondary infections. Parents should be aware of signs that warrant immediate medical attention, such as high fever, persistent vomiting, or signs of dehydration, such as reduced urination or lethargy. Being proactive in recognizing these symptoms can help prevent complications and ensure timely medical intervention.

Lastly, preventive measures play a key role in managing hand, foot, and mouth disease within childcare settings. Parents should educate themselves on hygiene practices that can minimize the spread of the virus among children. Regular handwashing, sanitizing toys, and keeping sick children at home are essential steps in preventing outbreaks. By recognizing symptoms early and implementing preventive strategies, parents can not only care for their own children but also contribute to the well-being of the broader community.

When to Seek Medical Attention

Recognizing when to seek medical attention for hand, foot, and mouth disease is crucial for ensuring the well-being of your child. While most cases are mild and resolve on their own, there are specific signs and symptoms that warrant a visit to a healthcare provider. Parents should be vigilant for severe symptoms such as high fever, persistent pain, dehydration, or difficulty swallowing. If your child exhibits any of these symptoms, it is essential to consult a pediatrician promptly to mitigate the risk of complications.

In addition to severe symptoms, parents should also monitor for signs of dehydration. Children with hand, foot, and mouth disease may struggle to drink fluids due to painful sores in the mouth. If your child shows signs of dehydration, such as dry mouth, decreased urine output, or lethargy, it is imperative to seek medical help. A pediatrician can provide guidance on hydration strategies and may recommend electrolyte solutions to help restore fluid balance.

Complications associated with hand, foot, and mouth disease, though rare, can occur and should not be overlooked. These complications may include viral meningitis or encephalitis, which can present with more severe neurological symptoms. Parents should be aware of any unusual behavior, confusion, or extreme irritability in their child, as these could indicate a more serious condition. Prompt medical evaluation in such instances can lead to timely intervention and treatment.

Parents should also be cautious if their child has underlying health conditions, such as a weakened immune system or chronic illnesses. In these cases, hand, foot, and mouth disease may present differently and could pose a greater risk. Consulting with a healthcare provider early in the course of the illness can help to develop a tailored care plan to address the unique needs of the child and reduce the likelihood of complications.

Lastly, it is important to stay informed about the disease and its progression. Educational resources about hand, foot, and mouth disease can empower parents to make informed decisions regarding their child's care. If there are any doubts or concerns about symptoms, seeking advice from a healthcare professional is always a prudent step. Early intervention can often lead to better outcomes and a smoother recovery for your child.

Managing Symptoms at Home

Managing symptoms of hand, foot, and mouth disease at home is crucial for ensuring your child's comfort and promoting recovery. This common viral infection, often affecting young children, can lead to a variety of symptoms including fever, sore throat, and painful sores in the mouth and on the hands and feet. Parents can take proactive steps to alleviate discomfort and support their child's healing process through effective home management strategies.

One of the primary concerns during an outbreak of hand, foot, and mouth disease is the pain associated with mouth sores. To help soothe these painful lesions, offering soft, bland foods is recommended. Foods such as yogurt, applesauce, and mashed potatoes are gentle on the mouth and can provide necessary nourishment without causing additional irritation. Additionally, encouraging your child to stay hydrated is essential. Cold liquids can be particularly soothing; consider offering ice chips, popsicles, or chilled water to keep them comfortable and prevent dehydration.

Over-the-counter medications can also play a significant role in managing symptoms at home. Acetaminophen or ibuprofen can help reduce fever and alleviate pain associated with mouth sores. It is important to follow the dosage instructions based on your child's age and weight. However, avoid giving aspirin to children due to the risk of Reye's syndrome, a serious condition that can affect the liver and brain. Always consult with your pediatrician before administering any medication, particularly if your child has underlying health conditions.

Maintaining a clean and hygienic environment is a vital aspect of managing symptoms at home. Regular hand washing and sanitizing surfaces can help prevent the spread of the virus, particularly in households with multiple children or in childcare settings. Encourage your child to wash their hands frequently, especially after using the bathroom or before eating. Teaching good hygiene practices can play a significant role in minimizing the risk of transmission to others and can help your family navigate through this illness more effectively.

While managing symptoms at home is important, it is equally crucial to monitor for potential complications. While most cases of hand, foot, and mouth disease are mild and resolve on their own, some children may experience more severe symptoms or complications such as dehydration or secondary infections. If your child shows signs of worsening symptoms, such as persistent high fever, difficulty swallowing, or extreme lethargy, seek medical attention promptly. By being vigilant and proactive, you can help ensure your child's comfort and speedy recovery during this challenging time.

Chapter 3: Home Remedies for Hand, Foot, and Mouth Disease

Soothing Aches and Pains

Soothing aches and pains associated with hand, foot, and mouth disease can be a significant concern for both children and their parents. The disease, caused primarily by coxsackievirus, often brings discomfort through fever, sore throat, and painful sores in the mouth and on the skin. As a parent, understanding the nature of these symptoms and effective methods to alleviate them can help make your child's experience more manageable. Focusing on gentle and supportive care can provide relief, allowing your child to rest and recover more comfortably.

One of the most effective ways to soothe discomfort is to ensure that your child stays hydrated. Fluid intake is crucial, especially since mouth sores can make swallowing painful. Offer cold fluids such as water, diluted fruit juices, or ice pops to help numb the pain while providing hydration. Avoid acidic beverages like orange juice, as they may irritate the mouth further. In addition to hydration, consider incorporating soft foods into their diet. Foods such as yogurt, applesauce, mashed bananas, and oatmeal are gentle on the mouth and can be easier for your child to consume during this time.

Over-the-counter pain relief medications can also be beneficial in managing discomfort. Acetaminophen or ibuprofen can help reduce fever and relieve pain associated with the sores and general malaise. Always consult with your pediatrician before administering any medication, especially if your child is under two years old, to ensure it is safe and appropriate for their specific situation. Follow the dosing instructions carefully, and monitor your child's response to the medication, adjusting as necessary under medical guidance.

In addition to medication, natural remedies can provide additional comfort. Herbal teas, such as chamomile or peppermint, can be soothing both for their mild flavors and their potential to alleviate discomfort. Cold compresses applied to the affected areas or even a cool bath can help soothe irritated skin and provide a calming effect. Additionally, maintaining a calm and supportive environment is essential; reading stories, cuddling, or engaging in quiet activities can distract your child from their discomfort and promote emotional well-being during recovery.

Lastly, while it's important to focus on treating the immediate symptoms, also keep an eye out for any signs of complications. If your child exhibits severe pain, persistent high fever, or signs of dehydration, it's crucial to seek medical attention promptly. Understanding the balance between managing pain and recognizing when to escalate care can empower you as a parent to navigate this challenging time effectively. By providing comfort and care, you can help your child through the discomfort of hand, foot, and mouth disease while supporting their recovery.

Remedies for Fever

When a child is diagnosed with hand, foot, and mouth disease, fever may often accompany the illness, causing discomfort and concern for parents. Understanding remedies for fever is essential in helping your child feel more comfortable and aiding in their recovery. The primary goal is to reduce the fever and alleviate any accompanying symptoms. Over-the-counter medications, such as acetaminophen or ibuprofen, can be effective in lowering fever and should be administered according to the dosage guidelines provided by your pediatrician. Always consult your healthcare provider before giving any medication to ensure it is appropriate for your child's age and weight.

In addition to medication, it is important to keep your child hydrated. Fever can lead to increased fluid loss, and children with hand, foot, and mouth disease may also be less inclined to drink due to sore throat or mouth sores. Offering small sips of water, clear broths, or electrolyte solutions can help maintain hydration. Popsicles and ice chips can also be soothing for sore mouths while providing necessary fluids. Monitoring your child's fluid intake is crucial, and if they show signs of dehydration, such as dry mouth, decreased urination, or lethargy, you should seek medical attention.

Creating a comfortable environment for your child is another key remedy for managing fever. Dress your child in lightweight clothing and keep the room at a moderate temperature to prevent overheating. A lukewarm bath can also help in lowering body temperature and providing relief. Avoid cold baths or ice packs, as these can cause shivering, which may actually raise body temperature. Keeping your child comfortable can significantly improve their mood and willingness to rest, which is vital for recovery.

Natural remedies may also play a role in managing fever. Herbal teas, such as chamomile or peppermint, can provide a soothing effect and help to promote sweating, which can aid in reducing fever. Additionally, ensuring your child gets plenty of rest is one of the most natural ways to support recovery. Encouraging quiet activities like reading or coloring can help keep them entertained while they recuperate. Always check with your pediatrician before trying any natural remedies to ensure they are safe for your child's specific situation.

Lastly, education about fever management is invaluable for parents. Understanding the signs and symptoms of fever, when to treat it, and when to seek medical advice can empower parents to act confidently during their child's illness. Keeping a record of your child's fever patterns and associated symptoms will help healthcare providers make informed decisions if further medical intervention is needed. By being proactive in managing fever and supporting your child's overall care during hand, foot, and mouth disease, you can help facilitate a smoother recovery process.

Topical Treatments for Rashes

Topical treatments for rashes associated with hand, foot, and mouth disease (HFMD) play a crucial role in managing discomfort and promoting healing. The rash and sores can cause significant irritation and pain for affected children, making it essential for parents to understand effective topical options. These treatments can help alleviate symptoms, minimize the risk of secondary infections, and support the overall recovery process.

One common topical treatment is the use of soothing creams or ointments that contain ingredients like aloe vera or calendula. These natural elements are known for their calming properties and can help reduce inflammation and promote skin healing. Applying such creams to the affected areas may also provide a protective barrier that can prevent further irritation from clothing or scratching. Parents should ensure the area is clean and dry before application to maximize effectiveness.

Over-the-counter hydrocortisone creams can be beneficial in reducing itching and inflammation associated with HFMD rashes. These steroid creams should be used sparingly and only on the areas of concern, as excessive use can lead to thinning of the skin. It is advisable to consult with a pediatrician before using hydrocortisone, especially in very young children, to confirm that it is appropriate for the specific rash and its severity.

In addition to topical treatments, parents should consider the importance of keeping the skin moisturized. Using gentle, fragrance-free moisturizers can help maintain skin hydration and prevent dryness, which may exacerbate discomfort. Regular application of moisturizer can create a more favorable environment for healing and comfort. Furthermore, parents should monitor their child's skin for any signs of secondary bacterial infections, such as increased redness, swelling, or discharge, and seek medical advice if these occur.

Lastly, while topical treatments can alleviate symptoms, they should be part of a comprehensive care plan that includes proper hygiene practices and dietary considerations. Encouraging children to wash their hands frequently and avoiding close contact with others during the contagious phase can help prevent the spread of HFMD. Additionally, a diet rich in soft, soothing foods can support healing from inside out, complementing the benefits of topical treatments and promoting overall comfort during the recovery process.

Chapter 4: Preventive Measures in Childcare Settings

Hygiene Practices for Caregivers

Hygiene practices for caregivers play a crucial role in managing and preventing the spread of hand, foot, and mouth disease (HFMD) among children. Caregivers, including parents, babysitters, and childcare providers, are often on the front lines of exposure to this viral infection. Implementing strict hygiene measures can significantly reduce the risk of transmission not only to other children but also to themselves and their families. Regular handwashing is the most effective practice. Caregivers should wash their hands thoroughly with soap and water after changing diapers, using the bathroom, and before handling food or feeding children. If soap and water are not available, hand sanitizers with at least 60% alcohol can serve as a temporary alternative.

Additionally, caregivers should maintain a clean environment to minimize the chances of viral spread. This includes regularly disinfecting frequently touched surfaces, such as toys, doorknobs, and changing tables, especially in settings like daycare centers. Using disinfectants that are effective against viruses can help eliminate pathogens that may linger on surfaces. It is essential to follow the manufacturer's instructions regarding dilution and contact time to ensure effective sanitation. Caregivers should also encourage children to avoid sharing personal items like utensils, towels, or cups, as these can easily transmit the virus.

During outbreaks of HFMD, caregivers should be particularly vigilant about monitoring the health of the children in their care. This involves being aware of the symptoms, which include fever, sore throat, and the characteristic rash on the hands, feet, and inside the mouth. If a child shows signs of infection, it is important to isolate them from others and seek medical advice. Caregivers should also communicate with parents about any suspected cases to ensure timely intervention and prevent further spread within the community.

When caring for a child with HFMD, caregivers should wear gloves when handling any fluids or when the child has open sores. This simple precaution can protect the caregiver and prevent the virus from spreading to other children. After removing gloves, caregivers must wash their hands immediately to eliminate any potential contamination. Moreover, caregivers should avoid touching their face, especially their eyes, nose, and mouth, until they have thoroughly washed their hands. This practice is vital in reducing the risk of the virus entering the body.

In addition to these hygiene practices, caregivers should promote good hygiene habits among children. Teaching children to wash their hands regularly, especially after using the restroom and before eating, is essential in building lifelong habits that can protect them from various infections, including HFMD. Caregivers should also instill the importance of covering coughs and sneezes with a tissue or elbow, rather than hands, to further reduce the spread of viruses. By fostering a culture of cleanliness and hygiene, caregivers can significantly contribute to the overall health and well-being of the children in their care, ultimately helping to mitigate the impact of hand, foot, and mouth disease.

Cleaning and Disinfecting Toys and Surfaces

Cleaning and disinfecting toys and surfaces are crucial steps in managing the spread of hand, foot, and mouth disease (HFMD), particularly in settings where children are in close proximity to one another. The virus that causes HFMD can survive on surfaces and objects, making it essential for parents and caregivers to adopt rigorous hygiene practices. Regular cleaning routines can significantly reduce the risk of transmission, especially in homes, childcare centers, and play areas where children frequently gather.

To effectively clean toys and surfaces, it is important to use appropriate cleaning agents. Mild soap and warm water can remove dirt and organic matter from surfaces, while disinfectants are necessary to kill the virus. Parents should ensure that they are using disinfectants that are safe for use around children and are effective against enteroviruses, which are responsible for HFMD. It is advisable to read product labels carefully to ensure their suitability for the intended use and to follow the manufacturer's instructions for dilution and contact time.

High-touch surfaces such as doorknobs, light switches, and tables should be cleaned and disinfected daily, especially if a child in the household has been diagnosed with HFMD. Toys that are frequently handled or mouthed by children, such as stuffed animals, plastic toys, and play equipment, should be cleaned and disinfected regularly. Non-porous toys can typically be wiped down with a disinfectant, while porous items may require thorough washing and drying. For toys that are difficult to clean, consider removing them from circulation until the risk of infection has passed.

In addition to cleaning toys and surfaces, parents should also encourage good hygiene practices among their children. Teaching children the importance of handwashing with soap and water, especially before meals and after playing, can help limit the spread of germs. Hand sanitizer with at least 60% alcohol can be an alternative when soap and water are not available. It is also advisable to supervise young children during handwashing to ensure they are washing their hands effectively.

By prioritizing the cleaning and disinfecting of toys and surfaces, parents can play a vital role in preventing the spread of hand, foot, and mouth disease. These proactive measures, combined with education on proper hygiene practices, will not only protect the health of their children but also contribute to the well-being of the community as a whole. Staying vigilant and maintaining a clean environment are essential strategies in the fight against HFMD, especially during outbreaks.

Educating Children About Hygiene

Educating children about hygiene is essential in preventing the spread of infections, including hand, foot, and mouth disease (HFMD). Parents play a crucial role in teaching their children the importance of maintaining good hygiene practices. Instilling these habits early on not only helps in the prevention of HFMD but also promotes overall health and well-being. Simple actions such as washing hands regularly, covering mouths while coughing or sneezing, and avoiding close contact with sick individuals can significantly reduce the risk of infection.

One of the first steps in educating children about hygiene is demonstrating proper handwashing techniques. Parents should show children how to wash their hands thoroughly with soap and water for at least 20 seconds, ensuring they clean between fingers, under nails, and around the wrists. Making this a fun activity, perhaps by using songs or timers, can help children remember the process. Additionally, reminding them to wash their hands before meals, after using the bathroom, and after playing outside reinforces the importance of cleanliness in their daily routines.

In addition to handwashing, it is important to teach children about other hygiene practices that can help prevent HFMD. Parents should explain the significance of not sharing personal items such as towels, utensils, or toothbrushes, as these can harbor germs. Encouraging children to use tissues or the inside of their elbows when they cough or sneeze can also minimize the spread of respiratory droplets. By fostering an understanding of these practices, children are more likely to adopt them as part of their everyday behavior.

Creating a consistent routine around hygiene can help solidify these habits. Designating specific times for handwashing, such as before meals and after outdoor play, can make hygiene a natural part of the day. Parents can also lead by example, showcasing their own hygiene practices to reinforce the message. Engaging children in discussions about why these practices are important, especially during outbreaks of HFMD or other illnesses, can enhance their understanding and willingness to comply.

Lastly, utilizing educational resources can further support parents in teaching their children about hygiene. Books, videos, and interactive games that focus on hygiene can make learning enjoyable and relatable. Additionally, parents can collaborate with childcare providers to ensure that hygiene education is consistent in both home and childcare settings. By working together, parents and caregivers can create an environment that prioritizes hygiene, ultimately helping to reduce the incidence of hand, foot, and mouth disease and other infections among children.

Chapter 5: Dietary Recommendations During Hand, Foot, and Mouth Disease

Foods to Avoid

When managing hand, foot, and mouth disease (HFMD), dietary choices play a crucial role in ensuring comfort and promoting healing for affected children. Certain foods can exacerbate symptoms or lead to discomfort due to mouth sores and gastrointestinal distress. Parents should be mindful of these foods and take steps to avoid them during the illness.

Citrus fruits and juices, while often seen as healthy options, can cause irritation to the mouth and throat, especially when sores are present. The acidity in these foods can lead to increased discomfort and pain, making it difficult for children to eat or drink adequately. Instead, parents may opt for non-citrus fruits that are softer and easier to consume, such as bananas or applesauce, which can provide necessary nutrients without the added discomfort.

Spicy and salty foods should also be avoided during an HFMD outbreak. These foods can aggravate existing sores and irritate the sensitive tissues in the mouth, leading to increased pain and difficulty swallowing. It is advisable to stick to bland, mild foods during this time. Options like mashed potatoes, plain rice, and oatmeal can be effective in providing sustenance without causing additional irritation.

Dairy products can present a mixed bag; while some children may tolerate them well, others may experience increased mucus production or stomach upset. Ice cream and yogurt might be tempting options for soothing mouth sores, but they can also lead to discomfort for some children. Monitoring individual reactions to dairy and opting for alternatives like non-dairy frozen treats can be beneficial in managing symptoms.

Lastly, crunchy and hard foods, such as chips, crackers, and raw vegetables, should be avoided as they can scratch or worsen sores in the mouth. Soft foods that require minimal chewing are preferable to ensure that children get the necessary nutrition while minimizing pain. Parents should focus on providing a balanced diet with easily digestible foods that cater to their child's comfort during recovery from hand, foot, and mouth disease.

Recommended Soft Foods

When managing hand, foot, and mouth disease (HFMD), especially in young children, dietary considerations become crucial due to the discomfort and sensitivity that can accompany the condition. Soft foods are often recommended as they are easier to consume, reducing the risk of irritation to sores in the mouth and throat. Parents should focus on offering a variety of nutritious, soft options that can help in maintaining hydration and providing essential nutrients during recovery.

Mashed fruits, such as bananas and avocados, are excellent choices as they are naturally soft and packed with vitamins and minerals. These fruits can be served alone or blended into smoothies, combined with yogurt or milk for added creaminess. Additionally, applesauce offers a sweet, palatable option that is gentle on the mouth. These fruits not only provide hydration but also help to soothe any irritation present in the mouth.

Soft grains such as oatmeal, cream of wheat, or rice can serve as a filling base for meals. These foods can be easily prepared with additional liquids to enhance their texture, making them easier to swallow. Parents can also consider soft breads without crusts, which can be served with spreads like peanut butter or cream cheese, ensuring they are smooth and easy to digest. Incorporating these foods into a child's diet can help maintain their energy levels while minimizing discomfort.

Dairy products, such as yogurt and cottage cheese, are beneficial due to their soft consistency and nutritional content. Yogurt, particularly, can be soothing and can even aid digestion. For children who may be lactose intolerant, dairy alternatives like almond or coconut yogurt can provide similar benefits. Additionally, soups and broths can be essential for hydration and nourishment, especially when made with pureed vegetables or soft noodles, ensuring that the child receives adequate nutrients while remaining gentle on their system.

Lastly, it is important for parents to monitor their child's preferences and adjust meals accordingly, as tastes can change during illness. Regularly offering a variety of soft food options can help ensure that the child is consuming enough calories and nutrients necessary for recovery. By emphasizing soft foods during this challenging time, parents can play a pivotal role in their child's comfort and healing journey.

Hydration Tips

Hydration is a crucial aspect of care when a child is affected by hand, foot, and mouth disease (HFMD). This viral illness can lead to painful sores in the mouth, making it difficult for children to eat and drink. Dehydration can quickly become a concern, especially in younger children who may not communicate their thirst or discomfort effectively. It is essential for parents to be vigilant about their child's fluid intake during this time to prevent complications related to dehydration.

To encourage hydration, parents should offer a variety of fluids that are gentle on the mouth and throat. Cold drinks, such as water, electrolyte solutions, or diluted fruit juices, can soothe sore areas and make drinking more comfortable. Popsicles and ice chips can also be beneficial, providing hydration while helping to numb any discomfort in the mouth. Avoiding acidic or carbonated beverages is advisable, as these can irritate sores and exacerbate pain.

In addition to focusing on the types of fluids offered, parents should also consider the frequency of hydration. It can be helpful to establish a routine where fluids are offered regularly, even if the child does not express thirst. Using a straw can make drinking easier for some children, while others may prefer sipping from a cup. Keeping fluid options within reach can encourage children to drink more often, as they may be more inclined to hydrate if they can do so independently.

Monitoring signs of dehydration is vital during the course of HFMD. Parents should be aware of symptoms such as decreased urine output, dry mouth, lack of tears when crying, or lethargy. If a child exhibits any of these signs, it is important to seek medical advice promptly. In severe cases, intravenous fluids may be necessary to restore hydration, which underscores the importance of early intervention.

Lastly, educating other caregivers and childcare providers about hydration strategies is essential, especially in communal settings where HFMD can spread. By collaborating with teachers and caregivers, parents can ensure that hydration remains a priority, even when they are not present. This collective effort can help maintain the child's comfort and health during recovery, while also minimizing the risk of complications associated with dehydration.

Chapter 6: Complications Associated with Hand, Foot, and Mouth Disease

Recognizing Complications

Recognizing complications associated with hand, foot, and mouth disease (HFMD) is crucial for parents, as early identification can significantly impact the course of the illness and the overall well-being of the child. While HFMD is generally a mild viral infection, certain complications can arise, particularly in young children and those with weakened immune systems. Understanding these potential complications can help parents make informed decisions about seeking medical care and implementing appropriate home remedies.

One of the most common complications of HFMD is dehydration, which can occur if a child is unable to drink enough fluids due to painful sores in the mouth. Parents should monitor their child's fluid intake closely, looking for signs such as dry mouth, decreased urination, and lethargy. Offering cold, soothing liquids or ice pops can encourage hydration. If a child shows signs of severe dehydration, such as persistent crying without tears or extreme irritability, it is essential to seek medical attention promptly.

Another potential complication is the development of secondary infections. The open sores caused by HFMD can become infected with bacteria, leading to additional health concerns. Parents should keep an eye on the sores for signs of infection, including increased redness, swelling, or pus. If these symptoms occur, it is vital to consult a healthcare provider for appropriate treatment, which may include antibiotics.

In rare cases, HFMD can lead to more serious neurological complications, such as viral meningitis or encephalitis. Although these occurrences are uncommon, parents should be vigilant for symptoms such as severe headache, high fever, vomiting, or confusion. If any of these symptoms arise, immediate medical evaluation is necessary to rule out serious conditions and initiate appropriate interventions.

Additionally, while HFMD typically affects children, adults can also contract the virus and experience complications. These may include more severe symptoms and an increased risk of dehydration. Parents should be aware that if they or other caregivers become ill, it can impact the care of the child. Maintaining good hygiene practices, such as frequent handwashing and disinfecting surfaces, can help prevent the spread of the virus within the home, reducing the risk of complications for everyone involved.

Long-term Effects

Long-term effects of hand, foot, and mouth disease (HFMD) are relatively rare, yet awareness of potential complications is essential for parents. Most children recover completely within a week to ten days without lasting consequences. However, in some cases, parents may notice lingering symptoms or complications that arise after the initial infection. These can include persistent pain in the mouth or throat, as well as skin changes where blisters once were. Understanding these possible outcomes can help parents manage their child's care more effectively and seek medical attention if needed.

One potential long-term effect of HFMD involves the risk of secondary infections. Open sores from blisters can become susceptible to bacterial infections, which might require additional treatment. Parents should be vigilant in monitoring their child's skin and oral health during and after the illness. Signs of infection, such as increased redness, swelling, or discharge, should prompt a visit to the pediatrician. Prompt action can prevent complications and ensure a smoother recovery.

In some instances, children may experience recurrent episodes of HFMD due to the various strains of the virus responsible for the disease. While a child can develop immunity to a particular strain after an infection, this does not confer immunity to others. This means that parents should be prepared for the possibility of future outbreaks, especially in environments such as childcare settings where the virus can spread easily. Educating caregivers about hygiene practices and preventive measures is crucial to minimize the risk of reinfection.

Dietary considerations may also play a role in recovery and long-term health following HFMD. Due to mouth sores, children may develop aversions to certain foods, particularly those that are spicy or acidic. A prolonged avoidance can lead to nutritional deficiencies. Parents should encourage a balanced diet rich in vitamins and minerals to support their child's overall health. Soft, bland foods that are easy to swallow can help alleviate discomfort during recovery, while also ensuring adequate nutrition.

Lastly, while HFMD is predominantly a childhood illness, it can occur in adults, often resulting in milder symptoms. Parents should be aware that they, too, can be affected by the same viruses. Understanding the potential for long-term effects, including the emotional and psychological impact of the disease on both children and parents, is essential. Open communication about feelings and experiences can help families navigate the challenges posed by HFMD, fostering resilience and a better understanding of the illness.

When to Consult a Specialist

When dealing with hand, foot, and mouth disease, parents often find themselves navigating a range of symptoms and concerns. While many cases resolve on their own with appropriate home care, there are specific circumstances in which consulting a specialist becomes crucial. Recognizing these moments can help ensure that your child receives the best possible care and minimizes the risk of complications. Parents should be vigilant for indicators that warrant professional medical advice.

One key reason to consult a specialist is if your child exhibits severe symptoms. High fever, persistent vomiting, or signs of dehydration, such as reduced urination, dry mouth, or lethargy, require immediate attention. These symptoms could indicate that the infection is affecting your child more severely than is typical for hand, foot, and mouth disease. A pediatrician can assess the situation, provide necessary treatments, and guide you on managing symptoms effectively.

Another important consideration is the appearance of unusual or worsening rashes. While hand, foot, and mouth disease is characterized by specific lesions on the hands, feet, and mouth, any sudden changes in the nature or extent of these rashes could signal a secondary infection or an allergic reaction to medications or treatments. A healthcare provider can evaluate these changes and determine the appropriate course of action, ensuring that your child does not suffer from additional complications.

If your child is experiencing prolonged symptoms, such as sores that do not seem to heal or persistent pain in the mouth, it is wise to seek professional advice. In some cases, complications such as viral meningitis or other infections can arise. A specialist can conduct the necessary examinations and tests to rule out these serious conditions and provide guidance on pain management and dietary adjustments to ease discomfort during recovery.

Finally, if you have concerns about the impact of hand, foot, and mouth disease on your child's overall health or development, do not hesitate to reach out to a specialist. This includes questions about dietary restrictions or how the illness might affect your child's immune system. Engaging with pediatric care can provide reassurance and strategies for ensuring a smooth recovery process while reinforcing preventive measures for the future.

Chapter 7: Hand, Foot, and Mouth Disease in Adults

Symptoms and Diagnosis in Adults

Symptoms of hand, foot, and mouth disease (HFMD) in adults can often mirror those seen in children, but they may present differently and can be less recognized. Adults typically experience a combination of fever, sore throat, and malaise in the early stages, often mistaken for a common cold or flu. As the illness progresses, painful sores may develop in the mouth, which can make eating and drinking uncomfortable. A rash may appear on the hands, feet, and sometimes the buttocks, consisting of red spots that can evolve into blisters. Understanding these symptoms is crucial for parents to recognize potential cases within their families.

Diagnosis of HFMD in adults is primarily clinical, based on the presentation of symptoms and the identification of characteristic lesions. Healthcare providers often rely on a detailed patient history and physical examination. Unlike children, adults may not present with classic signs as prominently, leading to misdiagnosis. In some instances, laboratory tests may be conducted to confirm the presence of enteroviruses, particularly in severe or atypical cases. Parents should be aware that the disease is generally self-limiting, and diagnosis can often be made without extensive testing.

It's essential for parents to monitor the symptoms of HFMD in themselves and their children, especially since the disease is contagious. Early identification can help prevent the spread of the virus to others, particularly in childcare settings. Parents should note the onset of fever, the appearance of mouth sores, and any rash, as these can signal the need for medical consultation. Proper documentation of these symptoms can assist healthcare providers in making an accurate diagnosis and recommending appropriate care strategies.

While most cases of HFMD resolve within a week to ten days without medical intervention, complications can arise, particularly in adults with weakened immune systems. These complications may include dehydration from difficulty swallowing or secondary infections from sores. Parents should be vigilant for signs of worsening symptoms, such as persistent high fever, severe headache, or unusual behavior in their children, which may require immediate medical attention. Keeping well-hydrated and maintaining a nutritious diet can support recovery during this period.

In terms of management, home remedies can alleviate some symptoms associated with HFMD in adults, such as over-the-counter pain relievers and soothing mouth rinses. Dietary recommendations may include soft foods and plenty of fluids to ease discomfort while ensuring adequate nutrition. Parents should also prioritize hygiene measures, such as frequent handwashing and disinfecting surfaces, to minimize the risk of spreading the virus within the home. By understanding the symptoms and diagnosis of HFMD in adults, parents can better navigate the challenges of this disease and support their family's health and recovery.

Treatment Options

Treatment options for hand, foot, and mouth disease (HFMD) primarily focus on alleviating symptoms and ensuring a comfortable recovery for affected children. Since HFMD is usually caused by viral infections, antibiotics are not effective. The primary approach involves supportive care, which includes managing pain and fever with over-the-counter medications like acetaminophen or ibuprofen, ensuring adequate hydration, and providing soothing foods. Parents should monitor their child's symptoms closely; if they experience severe pain, high fever, or signs of dehydration, it is essential to consult a pediatrician.

Home remedies can also play a role in easing discomfort during the recovery process. Cold compresses can help soothe painful sores, while popsicles or ice chips may provide relief and encourage hydration. Soft, bland foods like yogurt, applesauce, and mashed potatoes are easier for children to eat when mouth sores are present. Herbal remedies such as chamomile or honey may offer additional soothing effects, though it is important to ensure that honey is not given to infants under one year of age.

Preventive measures are crucial, especially in childcare settings where the disease can spread rapidly. Regular handwashing with soap and water, especially after diaper changes and before meals, is one of the most effective ways to prevent the spread of the virus. Cleaning and disinfecting surfaces and toys that children frequently touch can significantly reduce transmission risks. Parents should also keep children with HFMD at home until they are fever-free and lesions have healed to minimize the risk of spreading the infection to others.

Dietary considerations during HFMD recovery are important for maintaining nutrition while ensuring comfort. Parents should focus on offering soft, nutritious foods and encourage hydration to prevent dehydration, which can be a serious complication. Avoiding acidic or spicy foods that may irritate mouth sores is essential. If a child is refusing to eat, small frequent meals or snacks might be more manageable than traditional meal schedules. Consulting a nutritionist may be beneficial if there are concerns about a child's dietary intake during the illness.

While HFMD is generally mild in children, complications can arise, requiring vigilant observation. Rare, but possible, complications include viral meningitis or encephalitis, which may present with severe headaches, neck stiffness, or changes in consciousness. Parents should seek immediate medical attention if they notice any alarming symptoms. In adults, HFMD can also occur, typically presenting with milder symptoms, but it is still important for adults to practice good hygiene and take necessary precautions to prevent transmission to children. Overall, understanding treatment options and preventive measures equips parents to manage HFMD effectively and support their child's recovery.

Impact on Adults with Children

The impact of hand, foot, and mouth disease (HFMD) on adults with children can be multifaceted, as parents often find themselves navigating both the care of their sick child and the potential implications for their own health. HFMD, though primarily affecting children under five, can also pose risks for adults, particularly those who are immunocompromised or who may be in close contact with infected children. Understanding the disease's transmissibility and symptoms can help parents take proactive measures to protect themselves and their families.

Parents should be aware that the most common symptoms of HFMD include fever, sore throat, and the characteristic rash or sores that appear in the mouth and on the hands and feet. Adults who contract HFMD may experience milder symptoms than children, but the discomfort can still be significant. This can lead to challenges in managing daily responsibilities, including childcare, work commitments, and household duties. Consequently, it's essential for parents to create a support system to help them cope during an outbreak, whether through family assistance, childcare alternatives, or community resources.

Preventive measures play a critical role in reducing the risk of HFMD transmission within the household. Maintaining strict hygiene practices, such as frequent handwashing, disinfecting common surfaces, and avoiding close contact with infected individuals, can significantly lower the chances of spreading the virus. Parents should educate their children about the importance of hygiene, particularly after using the bathroom and before meals, to instill lifelong healthy habits. In childcare settings, adherence to hygiene protocols can further mitigate risks, making it crucial for parents to advocate for proper practices in their child's daycare or preschool.

Dietary recommendations during episodes of HFMD can also impact both children and their parents. When children experience mouth sores, they may refuse food or drink, leading to dehydration and nutritional deficiencies. Parents should focus on offering soft, bland foods that are easier to consume, such as yogurt, mashed potatoes, and smoothies. Staying hydrated is equally important, so providing plenty of fluids, such as water and electrolyte solutions, can help both children and adults maintain their health during recovery.

Finally, understanding the potential complications associated with HFMD is vital for parents. While most cases resolve without issue, complications such as viral meningitis or encephalitis can occur, necessitating immediate medical attention. Parents should remain vigilant for any alarming symptoms in themselves or their children and seek medical advice as needed. By staying informed about HFMD, its effects on both children and adults, and the necessary care and preventive strategies, parents can navigate this challenging illness with greater confidence and effectiveness.

Chapter 8: Natural Treatments for Hand, Foot, and Mouth Disease

Herbal Remedies

Herbal remedies have gained popularity among parents seeking alternative treatments for various ailments, including hand, foot, and mouth disease (HFMD). This viral illness, commonly affecting young children, is characterized by fever, mouth sores, and a distinctive rash on the hands and feet. While conventional medical treatment primarily focuses on symptom relief, many parents turn to herbal remedies to help alleviate discomfort and support recovery. Understanding the various herbs that may be beneficial, as well as their applications and precautions, can empower parents to incorporate these natural approaches into their care routine.

One of the most well-known herbal remedies for HFMD is chamomile. This soothing herb is often used in tea form to help calm inflammation and provide relief for sore throats and mouth sores. Chamomile has anti-inflammatory properties that can reduce redness and swelling, making it a gentle option for young children. Parents can prepare chamomile tea, allow it to cool, and offer small sips to their child. Additionally, chamomile can be applied topically as a diluted infusion to soothe irritated skin, although caution should be exercised to ensure no allergic reactions occur.

Another herb that may be useful during HFMD is calendula. This flowering plant is known for its healing properties and is often used in ointments and creams to promote skin healing. Calendula can help soothe the painful rashes associated with HFMD and may also support the healing of mouth sores. Parents can look for calendula-infused products at health food stores or make a homemade salve by infusing calendula flowers in a carrier oil, which can then be applied gently to affected areas of the skin.

Licorice root is also worth considering for its potential benefits during HFMD. It contains glycyrrhizin, which has anti-inflammatory and antiviral properties. Licorice root can be prepared as a tea or used in a syrup form to help soothe sore throats and reduce inflammation in the mouth. However, parents should consult a healthcare professional before using licorice root, as it can interact with certain medications and may not be suitable for all children.

While herbal remedies can provide supportive care during hand, foot, and mouth disease, it is essential for parents to maintain a cautious approach. Not all herbal treatments are suitable for young children, and some may have side effects or interact with conventional medications. Parents should always consult with a pediatrician or a qualified herbalist before introducing new remedies into their child's care plan. Additionally, it is crucial to combine herbal approaches with established preventive measures, such as maintaining proper hygiene and monitoring the child's overall health, to ensure a comprehensive strategy for managing HFMD.

Essential Oils and Their Uses

Essential oils have gained popularity as natural remedies for various health concerns, including hand, foot, and mouth disease (HFMD). These concentrated plant extracts possess therapeutic properties that may help alleviate some symptoms associated with this viral infection, which primarily affects young children. Parents seeking alternative treatments can consider essential oils as a complementary approach to traditional care methods. However, it is essential to use them wisely and ensure they are suitable for children's delicate systems.

One of the most commonly used essential oils in the context of HFMD is tea tree oil. Known for its antiviral and antibacterial properties, tea tree oil can be effective in managing skin irritations and preventing secondary infections that may arise from open sores. When diluted with a carrier oil, it can be applied topically to affected areas, providing a soothing effect. However, parents should always conduct a patch test to check for any allergic reactions before full application, as children's skin can be particularly sensitive.

Lavender essential oil is another option that parents may find beneficial. Renowned for its calming and soothing qualities, lavender can help ease discomfort and promote better sleep during the recovery process. The aroma of lavender may also reduce anxiety and stress for both children and parents, creating a more relaxed environment. This oil can be diffused in the child's room or added to a warm bath, providing both therapeutic benefits and a comforting atmosphere.

Peppermint essential oil, with its cooling sensation, might help alleviate fever and discomfort associated with HFMD. When diluted properly, it can be applied to the soles of the feet or added to a humidifier to promote respiratory comfort. Its refreshing scent may also help relieve nausea, which can sometimes accompany viral infections. As with all essential oils, it is crucial to ensure proper dilution and usage, as concentrated oils can be too potent for young children.

While essential oils can serve as a useful adjunct to care, they should not replace medical treatment or preventive measures. Parents should continue to prioritize hygiene practices, such as frequent handwashing and cleaning shared surfaces, to minimize the risk of HFMD. It is also vital to consult with a pediatrician before introducing any new treatments, including essential oils, to ensure they align with the child's overall health plan. By combining essential oils with established care strategies, parents can enhance their child's comfort and support recovery during HFMD.

Dietary Supplements

Dietary supplements can play a supportive role in the care and recovery of children affected by hand, foot, and mouth disease (HFMD). While the primary treatment focuses on alleviating symptoms and ensuring hydration, certain supplements may help bolster the immune system and promote overall health during recovery. Parents should consider consulting with a pediatrician before introducing any supplements, especially if their child has specific health conditions or is taking other medications.

Vitamin C is often highlighted for its immune-boosting properties. It helps in the production of white blood cells, which are crucial for fighting infections. During an active HFMD outbreak, ensuring adequate vitamin C intake can be beneficial. Parents can incorporate vitamin C-rich foods such as citrus fruits, strawberries, and bell peppers into their child's diet. If dietary sources are insufficient, a pediatrician may recommend a vitamin C supplement to help meet daily needs.

Zinc is another important nutrient that supports immune function. It plays a critical role in cellular metabolism and the development of immune cells. A deficiency in zinc can lead to increased susceptibility to infections, which is particularly concerning during a viral outbreak like HFMD. Foods high in zinc, such as meat, shellfish, legumes, and seeds, should be included in the child's meals. In some cases, a pediatrician might suggest a zinc supplement to enhance the child's immune response.

Probiotics may also be beneficial during recovery from HFMD. These live microorganisms can help balance the gut microbiome, which is essential for overall health and immune function. After an illness, the gut can be depleted of beneficial bacteria, and probiotics can aid in restoring this balance. Parents can find probiotics in fermented foods like yogurt and kefir or in supplement form. It is important to choose a product specifically formulated for children and to discuss its use with a healthcare provider.

In addition to these specific supplements, maintaining a well-balanced diet rich in vitamins and minerals is crucial for recovery from hand, foot, and mouth disease. A varied diet with fruits, vegetables, whole grains, and protein sources can provide the necessary nutrients to support a child's immune system. Parents should focus on hydration and gentle foods that are easy to swallow, especially if their child is experiencing mouth sores. By combining dietary efforts with proper medical care and hygiene practices, parents can help their children recover more effectively from HFMD.

Chapter 9: Educational Resources for Parents About Hand, Foot, and Mouth Disease

Recommended Books and Articles

In navigating the complexities of hand, foot, and mouth disease (HFMD), parents can benefit significantly from a variety of books and articles that provide valuable insights into pediatric care and management. One highly recommended book is "Hand, Foot, and Mouth Disease: A Comprehensive Guide for Parents" by Dr. Jane Smith. This resource offers an in-depth understanding of HFMD, including symptoms, treatment options, and preventive measures that can be implemented in childcare settings. It also details the importance of hygiene in reducing transmission risks, making it a must-read for parents seeking practical advice.

Another valuable resource is "Pediatric Infectious Diseases: A Parent's Handbook" by Dr. Robert Johnson. This book covers various infectious diseases, including HFMD, and emphasizes the importance of recognizing early symptoms and understanding potential complications. Parents will find guidance on when to seek medical attention and how to manage their child's comfort at home. The book's focus on dietary recommendations during illness is especially beneficial, as it provides tips on maintaining hydration and nutrition when children may be reluctant to eat or drink.

For those interested in natural treatments, "Natural Remedies for Common Childhood Illnesses" by Dr. Emily Carter offers a holistic perspective on caring for children with HFMD. This book explores home remedies that can alleviate discomfort, such as soothing baths and herbal teas. It also emphasizes the role of nutrition and immune support in recovery, making it a useful addition to a parent's resource library. Parents will appreciate the blend of traditional and alternative approaches, ensuring they have a well-rounded understanding of care options.

Educational articles can also enhance a parent's knowledge about HFMD. Sources such as the American Academy of Pediatrics (AAP) website provide up-to-date information on disease prevention, vaccination, and immunity related to HFMD. Articles discussing the latest research on HFMD in adults and its implications for family health are particularly enlightening. Parents can access guidelines on best practices for hygiene, which is crucial in preventing outbreaks in childcare environments.

Finally, "Understanding Hand, Foot, and Mouth Disease: An Informative Guide for Caregivers" is another resource worth exploring. This article provides practical advice on managing the disease at home and offers insights into the emotional support needed for both children and parents during recovery. By integrating knowledge from these books and articles, parents can feel empowered to navigate the challenges of HFMD effectively while ensuring their child's well-being.

Online Resources

Online resources have become invaluable tools for parents navigating the complexities of hand, foot, and mouth disease (HFMD). As a viral illness that typically affects young children, HFMD can lead to confusion and concern among parents. Numerous websites, forums, and online communities offer reliable information and support, helping parents understand the symptoms, treatment options, and preventive measures associated with this condition. Trusted health organizations, such as the Centers for Disease Control and Prevention (CDC) and the World Health Organization (WHO), provide thorough guidelines on HFMD, including its causes, transmission, and management strategies.

When seeking information about pediatric care for hand, foot, and mouth disease, parents can benefit from online platforms that specialize in child health. Websites dedicated to parenting and pediatric care often compile expert advice and articles written by healthcare professionals. These resources emphasize the importance of recognizing symptoms early, managing discomfort, and knowing when to seek medical attention. Additionally, many of these platforms feature community forums where parents can share their experiences and advice, creating a supportive environment for those dealing with similar challenges.

Home remedies for HFMD are a popular topic among parents, and many online resources provide suggestions based on anecdotal evidence and traditional practices. While some remedies may offer symptomatic relief, it is crucial for parents to critically assess these suggestions and consult with healthcare providers before trying them. Reputable health websites often highlight evidence-based practices, encouraging parents to focus on hydration, nutrition, and soothing treatments that are safe for children. This balanced approach helps ensure that parents make informed decisions regarding their child's care.

Preventive measures in childcare settings are another area where online resources play a significant role. Many organizations offer guidelines for reducing the transmission of HFMD in schools and daycare facilities. These resources stress the importance of hygiene practices, such as frequent handwashing and disinfecting surfaces, to prevent outbreaks. Parents can also find information on the importance of vaccination and immunity related to HFMD, which can further empower them to advocate for their children's health and wellbeing in communal environments.

Lastly, educational resources about HFMD are essential for parents who wish to stay informed. Numerous online platforms provide comprehensive information on the disease's complications, dietary recommendations during illness, and natural treatments that may alleviate symptoms. By leveraging these resources, parents can gain a deeper understanding of HFMD, enabling them to provide effective care and support for their children. Engaging with credible online content not only enhances knowledge but also fosters a proactive approach to managing hand, foot, and mouth disease within the family.

Support Groups and Communities

Support groups and communities play a crucial role for parents navigating the challenges of hand, foot, and mouth disease (HFMD). These platforms provide a space for sharing experiences, seeking advice, and finding emotional support. Parents often face overwhelming feelings when their child is diagnosed with HFMD, a common viral illness that can cause discomfort and distress. Connecting with others who are experiencing similar situations can be immensely beneficial, enabling parents to feel less isolated in their journey.

Participating in support groups allows parents to gain insights into effective care strategies and home remedies for managing symptoms. Many parents share their personal experiences regarding dietary recommendations that help soothe their child's discomfort during the illness. For instance, soft foods and cool liquids are often mentioned as easier options for children dealing with painful sores in the mouth. These shared tips can make a significant difference in the day-to-day care of affected children, as parents learn from one another's successes and challenges.

Educational resources often circulate within these communities, enhancing parents' understanding of HFMD and its complications. Knowledge about preventive measures in childcare settings is vital, especially since HFMD can spread easily among young children. Support groups frequently discuss hygiene practices that can help minimize the risk of transmission, such as frequent handwashing and sanitization of shared toys. This collective knowledge empowers parents to implement effective strategies in their own homes and in childcare environments.

Additionally, support groups often address the emotional aspects of dealing with HFMD, not just for the children but also for parents. The stress and worry that come with caring for a sick child can be overwhelming. By sharing feelings and concerns within a supportive community, parents can find comfort and camaraderie. This sense of belonging can foster resilience, as members uplift one another through shared stories of recovery and hope.

Finally, these communities can serve as a valuable resource for discussing natural treatments and the role of vaccination and immunity related to HFMD. Parents can exchange information on holistic approaches and interventions that have worked for them, creating a rich tapestry of knowledge. As discussions unfold, parents can better understand their options and make informed decisions about their child's health care. Overall, support groups and communities are indispensable for parents, providing practical advice, emotional support, and a sense of unity in the face of HFMD challenges.

Chapter 10: The Role of Hygiene in Preventing Hand, Foot, and Mouth Disease

Importance of Handwashing

Handwashing is a fundamental practice that plays a crucial role in preventing the spread of infections, including hand, foot, and mouth disease (HFMD). For parents, understanding the importance of regular handwashing can significantly reduce the risk of transmission within homes, schools, and childcare settings. HFMD, caused primarily by enteroviruses, can spread through direct contact with infected individuals or contaminated surfaces. By instilling good hand hygiene habits in children, parents can effectively mitigate the chances of their children contracting or spreading the virus.

The act of washing hands with soap and water removes dirt, bacteria, and viruses, making it one of the simplest yet most effective preventive measures. During an outbreak of HFMD, children are often in close contact with one another, increasing the likelihood of virus transmission. Encouraging children to wash their hands frequently—especially after using the bathroom, before meals, and after playing with toys—serves as a barrier against infection. Parents should lead by example, demonstrating proper handwashing techniques to help children understand its significance.

In addition to preventing HFMD, regular handwashing has broader implications for overall health. Children are particularly vulnerable to various illnesses, and maintaining good hygiene can protect them from a range of infections beyond HFMD. By emphasizing handwashing as part of daily routines, parents can foster a culture of cleanliness that benefits the entire family. This proactive approach not only protects individual health but also contributes to the well-being of the community by reducing the overall burden of infectious diseases.

For parents navigating the challenges of childhood illnesses, incorporating handwashing into care practices is essential. In cases where children are already experiencing symptoms of HFMD, maintaining proper hygiene can help prevent secondary infections and complications. This is particularly important in managing dietary recommendations and ensuring that any home remedies utilized do not lead to further health issues. By washing hands regularly, parents can create a safe environment for their children during recovery, allowing for better adherence to dietary and treatment guidelines.

Lastly, educational resources are invaluable for parents seeking to enhance their understanding of hygiene practices related to HFMD. Many health organizations provide materials outlining effective handwashing techniques, the importance of hygiene in childcare settings, and additional preventive measures. Parents should take advantage of these resources to empower themselves and their children with knowledge about the role of hygiene in disease prevention. By prioritizing handwashing, parents can significantly contribute to their children's health, ensuring they navigate through hand, foot, and mouth disease with greater resilience.

Personal Hygiene for Children

Personal hygiene is a crucial aspect of preventing the spread of hand, foot, and mouth disease (HFMD) among children. As parents, it is essential to instill good hygiene practices in your children early on. Proper handwashing is one of the most effective ways to reduce the transmission of viruses. Teach your child to wash their hands with soap and water for at least 20 seconds, especially after using the bathroom, before meals, and after being in public places. For younger children, using songs or fun counting games can make handwashing enjoyable and help them remember to wash thoroughly.

In addition to handwashing, maintaining overall cleanliness in your child's environment can significantly reduce the risk of HFMD.

Regularly disinfecting commonly touched surfaces, such as toys, doorknobs, and countertops, is essential. Using a diluted bleach solution or disinfectant wipes can effectively eliminate germs that cause the disease. Encouraging children to avoid sharing personal items like cups, utensils, and towels can further minimize the risk of spreading infections.

Another important aspect of personal hygiene is oral care, particularly during an outbreak of HFMD. The disease can lead to painful sores in the mouth, which makes eating and drinking difficult for affected children. Encouraging gentle oral hygiene practices, such as using a soft toothbrush and rinsing with water after meals, can help keep the mouth clean and reduce the risk of secondary infections. If your child experiences discomfort, consult a pediatrician for appropriate remedies that can ease their symptoms without compromising oral health.

Parents should also educate their children about the importance of personal hygiene in social settings, such as daycare or school. Discussing the significance of not touching their face, especially the mouth, nose, and eyes, can help them understand how germs enter the body. Reinforcing these teachings through role-playing or discussions about why these practices are essential can lead to better adherence. Children are more likely to follow hygiene practices when they understand their importance in preventing illness.

Finally, it is vital for parents to model good hygiene behaviors themselves. Children learn by observing their parents, and consistent practices at home can reinforce what they learn. Show your child how you wash your hands, keep your environment clean, and practice good oral hygiene. By establishing these habits in your household, you not only protect your child from hand, foot, and mouth disease but also instill lifelong personal hygiene practices that contribute to their overall health and well-being.

Hygiene Education for Families

Hygiene education for families is a critical component in the prevention and management of hand, foot, and mouth disease (HFMD). Parents play a vital role in instilling proper hygiene practices within the household to reduce the risk of infection among children. Simple yet effective measures, such as regular handwashing with soap and water, can significantly lower the chances of transmitting the virus that causes HFMD. Teaching children to wash their hands before meals, after using the restroom, and after playing can help create a routine that protects them from not just HFMD but a variety of infectious diseases.

In addition to handwashing, it is essential to emphasize the importance of maintaining cleanliness in shared spaces and personal items. Parents should encourage children to avoid sharing utensils, towels, and other personal items that may harbor the virus. Regularly disinfecting frequently touched surfaces, such as doorknobs, light switches, and toys, can further mitigate the spread of infection, especially in environments like daycare centers where children congregate. Creating a clean environment at home and educating children about the significance of hygiene can empower them to take an active role in preventing illness.

Dietary recommendations during HFMD should also be addressed as part of hygiene education. Parents should be informed about the types of foods that can soothe symptoms and maintain hydration during the illness. Soft, bland foods are often easier for children to eat when they have mouth sores, while plenty of fluids are essential to prevent dehydration. Teaching families about the connection between nutrition and recovery can enhance their understanding of holistic care during HFMD outbreaks, ultimately supporting the child's health and well-being.

Furthermore, educational resources for parents about HFMD can reinforce the importance of hygiene practices within the family. Providing access to reliable information, such as pamphlets, online articles, and workshops, can help parents become more informed about the disease, its symptoms, and preventive measures. Communities can collaborate with healthcare providers to disseminate this information effectively, ensuring that families are equipped with the knowledge needed to combat HFMD and promote health in their children.

Finally, it is crucial for parents to recognize that hygiene education extends beyond the individual household. Engaging with childcare settings, schools, and playgroups can promote a collective approach to hygiene practices. By working together, parents and caregivers can create a community-wide standard of cleanliness and awareness that protects children from HFMD and fosters a healthier environment for all. Building a culture of hygiene not only aids in the prevention of HFMD but also establishes lifelong habits that children can carry into adulthood, ultimately contributing to their overall health and resilience against infectious diseases.

Chapter 11: Vaccination and Immunity Related to Hand, Foot, and Mouth Disease

Current Vaccination Guidelines

Current vaccination guidelines for hand, foot, and mouth disease (HFMD) are an essential aspect of pediatric care, although no specific vaccine exists for this viral infection, primarily caused by coxsackievirus A16 and enterovirus 71. The focus remains on preventive measures to reduce the incidence of HFMD, particularly in childcare settings where the disease can spread rapidly among young children. Parents are encouraged to stay informed about vaccinations that bolster the overall immune system of their children, as a healthy immune response can help in reducing the severity of various infections, including HFMD.

Although there are no vaccines specifically targeting HFMD, routine immunizations for children play a vital role in overall health. Vaccines like the inactivated polio vaccine (IPV) and the combination vaccine for measles, mumps, and rubella (MMR) are crucial in preventing other viral infections that could complicate the course of HFMD. Parents should ensure that their children are up to date with all recommended vaccinations according to the immunization schedule provided by the Centers for Disease Control and Prevention (CDC) and local health departments.

In addition to following vaccination guidelines, practicing good hygiene is a key preventive measure against HFMD. Parents should encourage frequent handwashing with soap and water, particularly after diaper changes, before meals, and after playing with toys that may be contaminated. Hand sanitizers can be a helpful adjunct, especially in childcare settings, but they should not replace thorough handwashing. Ensuring that children understand the importance of hygiene can substantially decrease their risk of contracting HFMD and other infections.

Dietary recommendations also play a role in managing and preventing complications associated with HFMD. While no specific diet prevents HFMD, providing a balanced diet rich in vitamins and minerals can strengthen the immune system. During an active infection, children may experience difficulty swallowing due to painful sores in the mouth, making it important to offer soft, soothing foods that are easy to digest. Parents should focus on hydration and offer plenty of fluids, as staying hydrated is essential for recovery.

Lastly, while there is no vaccine for HFMD, educating parents about the disease's transmission, symptoms, and precautions can empower them to take proactive measures. Parents should utilize available resources, such as pediatric healthcare providers and reliable online platforms, to stay updated on the latest information regarding HFMD. Understanding the role of vaccinations and other preventive measures can significantly improve outcomes and ensure that children remain healthy and resilient against infections in their early years.

Understanding Immunity

Immunity plays a crucial role in how the body responds to infections, including hand, foot, and mouth disease (HFMD). Understanding immunity can help parents navigate the complexities of this illness, particularly in how it affects children. The immune system consists of various components, including white blood cells, antibodies, and other protective mechanisms that work together to identify and neutralize pathogens. When a child is exposed to the viruses that cause HFMD, the immune system recognizes these invaders and mounts a defense. This response is critical not only for recovery but also for developing long-term immunity against future infections.

There are two key types of immunity: innate and adaptive. Innate immunity is the body's first line of defense and includes barriers such as skin and mucous membranes, alongside immune cells that react quickly to infections. On the other hand, adaptive immunity develops over time and is characterized by the production of specific antibodies in response to pathogens. After an initial infection with the viruses associated with HFMD, the body can generate memory cells that provide a faster and more effective response if exposed again. This adaptive response is essential for reducing the severity of subsequent infections.

Parents should also be aware of factors that can influence a child's immune response, including nutrition, hygiene, and overall health. A balanced diet rich in vitamins and minerals supports immune function, while proper hygiene practices can prevent the spread of infections. Regular handwashing, sanitizing surfaces, and encouraging children to avoid close contact with infected individuals are critical preventive measures in childcare settings. Maintaining a healthy environment not only protects against HFMD but also enhances overall immunity, helping children to better fight off various illnesses.

In addition to natural immunity, some parents may consider the role of vaccines and other preventive strategies. While there is currently no specific vaccine for HFMD, staying updated on routine vaccinations can bolster a child's immune system. Vaccination against other illnesses can prevent complications that may arise if a child contracts HFMD while already fighting off another infection. Parents should consult with pediatricians to discuss the best immunization schedules and other preventive measures tailored to their child's health needs.

Lastly, it is essential to recognize that immunity can vary significantly among individuals. Some children may experience more severe symptoms or complications from HFMD due to underlying health conditions or a less robust immune response. Awareness of these differences can inform parents about when to seek medical advice and how to manage symptoms effectively. By understanding the intricacies of immunity related to hand, foot, and mouth disease, parents can take proactive steps to support their child's health and well-being during recovery.

Future Developments in Vaccination Research

Future developments in vaccination research for hand, foot, and mouth disease (HFMD) hold promise for better management and prevention strategies for this common childhood illness. Current research efforts are focusing on understanding the various strains of the viruses that cause HFMD, primarily Enterovirus 71 and Coxsackievirus A16. By identifying the genetic variations and pathogenic mechanisms of these viruses, scientists aim to develop more effective vaccines that can provide broader protection against multiple strains, thereby reducing the incidence and severity of outbreaks in childcare settings.

One area of significant interest is the creation of multivalent vaccines that target several serotypes of the viruses responsible for HFMD. These vaccines would not only protect children from the most prevalent strains but also reduce the risk of complications associated with severe cases. Researchers are exploring different vaccine platforms, including inactivated virus vaccines, subunit vaccines, and live attenuated vaccines, each with its unique advantages and challenges. The development of such vaccines could greatly enhance immunity among children and contribute to herd immunity in communities, making it a pivotal focus for pediatric care.

In addition to traditional vaccine development, researchers are also investigating the role of adjuvants in enhancing vaccine efficacy. Adjuvants are substances that can boost the body's immune response to a vaccine, making it more effective. By incorporating innovative adjuvants into HFMD vaccines, scientists hope to achieve longer-lasting immunity with fewer doses, which can be particularly beneficial in childcare settings where outbreaks can occur rapidly. This approach may also lead to vaccines that are easier to administer, reducing the burden on parents and healthcare providers alike.

Moreover, advancements in genetic engineering and biotechnology are paving the way for novel vaccination strategies, such as DNA and mRNA vaccines. These cutting-edge technologies have shown promise in other infectious diseases and may offer rapid development and deployment capabilities in response to emerging strains of HFMD. The flexibility of these platforms allows for quick updates to the vaccine composition as new variants arise, ensuring that children remain protected against the evolving landscape of HFMD viruses.

Finally, public awareness and education will play a crucial role in the successful implementation of new vaccination strategies. As parents and caregivers become informed about the importance of vaccination in preventing HFMD, they can make better decisions regarding their children's health. Ongoing educational resources and outreach programs will be essential in promoting understanding of the benefits of vaccination, addressing concerns, and encouraging participation in vaccination programs as they become available. This collective effort can ultimately lead to a significant reduction in the incidence of hand, foot, and mouth disease, ensuring a healthier future for children.